Paleo Diet

The Ultimate Beginner's Guide To Paleo Diet Plan -
Proven Recipes To Lose Weight

(Paleo Diet Recipes For Beginners)

Julius Swanson

TABLE OF CONTENTS

Tomato-Okra Fry 1

Stirred Radish With Green Gram 3

Flour Infused Radish Leaves 5

Stirred Cucumber 7

Pumpkin With Dry Spices 10

Flour Infused Pumpkin 12

Stirred French Beans 15

French Beans In Coconut Pulp 17

Stirred French Beans With Potato 19

Veggie Omelet 21

Tender Milk Omelet 23

Masala Fresh Eggs 24

Egg-Lemon Sauce 27

Egg-Tomato Curry 28

Tomato Chicken 30

Boiled Chicken In Pink Stew 32

Chicken In Coriander-Spinach Stew 34

- Mushroom Infused Grilled Chicken 36
- Green Pomfrets 38
- Carrot Coconut Muffins 41
- Pumpkin Ice-Cream 42
- Strawberry Gateau 44
- Beetroot And Mustard Chips 46
- Roasted Kale Chips 47
- Parmesan Chips 48
- Devilled Fresh Eggs 49
- Cheesy Zucchini And Broccoli Soup 51
- Garlic Castilian Soup 53
- Dill And Leek Soup 55
- Grain-Free Vegan Mushroom Creamy Soup 57
- Vegan Gazpacho 59
- Vegan Creamy Broccoli Soup 61
- Mixed Greens Creamy Soup 63
- Tomato Soup 65

- Wholly Appetizing Mango Chia Seed Pudding 66
- Chocolaty Cocoa Mousse 67
- Exquisite Pumpkin Nut Butter Cup 69
- Tender Chocolate Silk Pie 71
- Crunchy Cinnamon Apple Chips 74
- Juice Popeye's Blueberry Smoothie 76
- Palatable Candied Pecans 78
- Crispy Balsamic Rosemary Roasted Vegetables 80
- Astonishingly Spiced And 82
- Stunning Eggplant Caponata 84
- Perfectly Sautéed Mushroom 86
- Sweetly Sautéed Radishes 87
- Gracefully Roasted Heirloom Carrots 89
- Intensely Blistered Beans With Crushed Almond 91
- Perplexing Cauliflower Couscous With Apricots And 93

Spring Chicken Salad 96

Raw Kale Salad 98

Creamed Spinach 100

Roasted Thyme Mushroom 102

Creamy Chicken Onion Soup............................. 104

Grand Pumpkin Soup 106

Mushroom Mussels Chowder 108

The Best Vegetable Soup 111

Turkey Potage 113

Grandma's Apple Ketchup 116

Coconut Mayonnaise 118

Paleo Salsa Verde 120

Sausage Casserole 121

Tangy Herb Frittata 125

Chicken Burrito 127

Salmon Cakes 129

Fish Tacos 131

Lemon Lobster Salad.. 133

Tropical Chicken Fingers 135

Slow Cooker Rustic Chicken Chili 137

Masala Chicken And Cauliflower Rice 139

Texan Bbq Meatballs 144

'Guilt-Free' Taco Pie 146

Classic Coconut Tapioca Pudding 150

Pumpkin Cookies 153

Balsamic Cremini Roast Beef 155

Coconut Milk Hot Chocolate 157

Banana Pumpkin Booster 158

Maple Date Brownies 159

Grilled Lemon Herb Lamb Chops 162

Pacific Passion Steak 164

Sour And Spicy Tuna 166

Authentic Chinese Shrimp 168

Aztec Fish Stew 170

Jamaican Ribs 172

Crackling Pork Chili 175

Bigos 177

Butter Chicken 179

Taro Chips 181

Salt Crackers 182

Bengali Almonds 183

The James' Secret Dill Pickles 185

Vermont Sweet Pecans 186

Tomato-Okra Fry

Ingredients:

1/2 tsp Coriander seed powder

1/2 tsp Mustard seeds

1/2 tsp Turmeric powder

1/2 tsp Asafetida

250 gm fresh tender Okra's

2 medium Potato

2 Tomatoes

2 Green Chilly

Instructions:

1. Clean the potato, peel off its skin and cut it into thin vertical strips.
2. Finely dice the tomatoes.

3. Wash the Okra and remove the hard stems, then cut it into small, thin wheels.
4. Finely chop the green chilly.
5. Heat the cooking oil in a pan.
6. Once the oil is hot, add the mustard seeds, asafetida and turmeric powder.
7. Once the mustard starts crackling, add the chopped chilly and tomatoes. Stir for a couple of minutes.
8. Then add the potato strips and stir till the potato becomes a bit red, then add the okra, coriander seed powder and salt.
9. Place a lid on the pan and let the okra cook for a few minutes.
10. Then remove the lid and stir well till all the moisture evaporates and you get a crispy okras. Serve while hot.

Stirred Radish With Green Gram

Ingredients:

1/2 tsp Turmeric powder

1/2 tsp Asafetida

2 -2 tbsp Cooking Oil

Salt to taste

2 fresh, tender Radishes

4 tbsp split Green Gram

2 green Chilly, finely diced

1/2 tsp Coriander seed powder

1/2 tsp Mustard seeds

Instructions:

1. Soak the split green grams for at least 5-7 hrs.
2. Wash the radish and finely dice it.
3. Heat the cooking oil in a pan.
4. Once the oil is hot, add the mustard seeds, asafetida and turmeric powder.
5. Once the mustard starts crackling, add the chilly followed by the soaked split green grams.
6. Stir for a couple of minutes and then add the diced radish. Sprinkle salt and coriander seed powder over the radish and stir well over a low flame.
7. Place a lid on the pan and let it cook.
8. Once the radish is cooked, remove the lid and continuously stir till the excess moisture evaporates.
9. Serve while hot.

Flour Infused Radish Leaves

Ingredients:

1/2 tsp Coriander seed powder

1/2 tsp Mustard seeds

1/2 tsp Turmeric powder

1/2 tsp Asafetida

2 -2 tbsp Cooking Oil

Salt to taste

2 bowl fresh, tender Radishes leaves

1 a cup of diced Radish

5-7 cloves of Garlic

2 green Chilly

Instructions:

1. Wash the radish leaves with water, drain the water and chop them.
2. Make a chilly-garlic paste.
3. Heat the cooking oil in a pan.
4. Once the oil is hot, add the mustard seeds, asafetida and turmeric powder.
5. Once the mustard starts crackling, add the chilly-garlic paste and stir for a minute.
6. Then add the diced radish to the pan and let it simmer for a couple of minutes.
7. Then add the radish leaves to the pan followed by the coriander seed powder and salt.
8. Place a lid over the pan and leave till the leaves are cooked.

9. Then remove the lid and stir over a low flame till the excess moisture evaporates.
10. Serve while hot.

Stirred Cucumber

Ingredients:

2-4 Curry leaves

1/2 tsp Mustard seeds

1/2 tsp Cumin seeds

1/2 tsp Asafetida

Salt to taste

2 -2 tbsp Cooking Oil

4 medium sized Cucumbers

2 tbsp split Bengal Gram

2 green Chilly, finely chopped

1/2 tsp Coriander seed powder

Instructions:

1. Soak the split bengal grams overnight
2. De-skin the cucumbers and finely dice them.
3. Heat the cooking oil in a pan.
4. Once the oil is hot, add the cumin seeds, mustard seeds, asafetida, chilly and curry leaves.
5. Once the cumin starts crackling, add the soaked bengal gram and stir for a couple of minutes.
6. Then add the finely diced cucumbers and coriander seed powder and salt.
7. Cover the pan with a lid and let it cook over a low flame for 2 minutes.
8. Then remove the lid and keep stirring till the excess moisture dries up.
9. Serve hot.

Pumpkin With Dry Spices

Ingredients:

1/2 tsp Poppy Seeds (*Khas Khas*)

1/2 tsp Cumin seeds

1/2 tsp Asafetida

1/2 tsp Turmeric powder

Salt to taste

2 -2 tbsp Cooking Oil

30 0 gm red Pumpkin

2 tbsp roasted Almonds, roughly grated

2 tbsp dried coconut, roughly grated

2 dried red chilly

1/2 tsp Fenugreek seeds

Instructions:

1. Peel off the skin from the pumpkin, also remove the seed and chop it into small bite size pieces.
2. Roast fenugreek seeds, poppy seeds, dried red chili and grated coconut, together in a pan for a couple of minutes. Then grind these ingredients into fine powder.
3. Heat the cooking oil in a pan.
4. Once the oil is hot, add the cumin seeds, asafetida and turmeric powder.
5. Once the cumin starts crackling, add the pumpkin to the pan followed by the dry spices powder we have created earlier.
6. Add salt to taste and cover with a lid.
7. Let it cook over steam for a few minutes, then remove the lid and keep stirring till the excess moisture dries up.
8. Serve hot.

Flour Infused Pumpkin

Ingredients:

2 green chili, finely chopped

1/2 tsp Mustard seeds

1/2 tsp Asafetida

1/2 tsp Turmeric powder

2 -2 tbsp Cooking Oil

Salt to taste

250 gm red Pumpkin

2 tbsp Chickpea flour

1/2 tsp coriander seed powder

Instructions:

1. Peel off the skin from the pumpkin, also remove the seed and chop it into small bite size pieces.
2. Heat the cooking oil in a pan.
3. Once the oil is hot, add the mustard seeds, asafetida, turmeric powder and chopped chili.
4. Once the mustard starts crackling, add pumpkin, coriander seed powder and salt. Stir for a while and then put a lid on the pan and let it simmer over a low flame.
5. Once it is cooked, remove the lid and sprinkle the chickpea flour in the pan, while continuously stirring the contents of the pan.
6. Once the flour is sprinkled, add 2 -2 tsp of cooking oil and then again stir till the excess moisture dries up.
7. Garnish with chopped coriander leaves and serve hot.

Stirred French Beans

Ingredients:

2-4 Curry Leaves

1/2 tsp Cumin seeds

1/2 tsp Asafetida

1/2 tsp Turmeric powder

2 -2 tbsp Cooking Oil

Salt to taste

250 gm fresh French Beans

2 green chilly finely chopped

1/2 tsp Cumin seed powder

1/2 tsp Coriander seed powder

2 -2 tsp Fresh Lemon Juice

Instructions:

1. Clean the french beans, and chop them into small pieces.
2. Boil 1 a liter water and put the beans in it, leave for 2 minutes.
3. Remove the beans and keep them in a strainer, so the excess water drains off.
4. Heat the cooking oil in a pan.
5. Once the oil is hot, add the curry leaves, cumin seeds, asafetida, turmeric powder and chilly.
6. Once the cumin starts crackling, add the french beans followed by the coriander seed powder, Cumin seeds powder and salt.
7. Keep stirring over a low flame till all the excess water dries off, then add the lemon juice, stir a few times and serve hot.

French Beans In Coconut Pulp

Ingredients:

2-4 Curry Leaves

2 tsp grated Ginger

1/2 tsp Cumin seeds

1/2 tsp Asafetida

1/2 tsp Turmeric powder

2 -2 tbsp Cooking Oil

Salt to taste

250 gm fresh French Beans

2 green chilly finely chopped

2 cup fresh Coconut Pulp, finely grated

2 dried red chilly finely chopped

Instructions:

1. Clean the french beans, and chop them into small pieces.
2. Heat the cooking oil in a pan.
3. Once the oil is hot, add the cumin seeds, asafetida, ginger and chilies.
4. Once the cumin starts crackling, add around 2 /4 rd of the grated coconut pulp, add salt to taste and keep stirring for 2-4 minutes.
5. Then add the french beans and turmeric powder to the pan, stir a bit and then cover the pan with a lid.
6. Remove the lid after 4-6 minutes and add the rest of the grated coconut pulp and stir till the excess moisture dries up.
7. Garnish with chopped coriander leaves and serve hot.

Stirred French Beans With Potato

Ingredients:

1/2 tsp Mustard seeds

1/2 tsp Cumin seeds

1/2 tsp Asafetida

1/2 tsp Turmeric powder

2 -2 tbsp Cooking Oil

Salt to taste

250 gm fresh French Beans

2 medium sized Potato, finely diced

2 medium sized Onion, finely diced

1/2 tsp Coriander seed powder

1/2 tsp red chili powder

Instructions:

1. Clean the french beans, and chop them into vertical thin strips.
2. Heat the cooking oil in a pan.
3. Once the oil is hot, add the cumin seeds, mustard seeds, turmeric and asafetida.
4. Once the mustard starts crackling, add onion and stir till it turns pink.
5. Then add potato and again keep stirring till it turns a bit red.
6. Then add the french beans, coriander seed powder and red chili powder.
7. Cover the pan with a lid and let it cook over a low flame for a few minutes.
8. Once it is cooked, remove the lid and stir till excess moisture dries up.
9. Garnish with fresh coriander leaves. Serve hot.

Veggie Omelet

Ingredients:

2 tbsp grated Green Capsicum

1/2 tsp green Chili paste

1/2 tsp Black Pepper powder

Salt to taste

2-4 tbsp Cooking Oil

4 Fresh Eggs

2 tbsp Green Peas

2 tbsp grated Onion

2 tbsp Tomato

Instructions:

1. Crack the fresh Eggs and remove the yolk from the egg whites and beat both separately. (add salt and black pepper

powder to the fresh Eggs while beating)
2. Then again mix the egg whites and yolks together once they are properly beaten.
3. Heat the cooking oil in a pan.
4. Once the oil is hot, add all the grated and diced veggies, salt and green chili paste to the pan and stir well for a couple of minutes.
5. Then add the fresh Eggs to the pan and cover the pan with a lid. (let it cook on medium heat).
6. Flit over the omelet to cook the other side. Serve hot.

Tender Milk Omelet

Ingredients:

Salt to taste

2 -2 tbsp Cooking Oil

2 Fresh Eggs

2 tbsp Milk

Instructions:

1. Crack the fresh Eggs into a bowl, add milk and salt to the fresh Eggs and beat them well.
2. Heat the cooking oil in a pan.
3. Once the oil is hot, pour in the beaten fresh Eggs to make the omelet.
4. The milk added makes the omelet juicy and tender.
5. Serve hot with a garnish of fresh Coriander leaves.

Masala Fresh Eggs

Ingredients:

4 tbsp grated fresh Coconut pulp

4 tbsp green Peas (boiled)

1/2 tsp Turmeric powder

1 tbsp chopped Coriander leaves

Salt to taste

2 -2 tbsp Cooking Oil

4 Fresh Eggs

2 tbsp Milk

2 medium sized Onions

1/2 tbsp green Chili paste

1 tsp Garlic paste

Instructions:

1. Crack the fresh Eggs into a bowl, add milk and salt to the fresh Eggs and beat them well.
2. Cut the Onions vertically into thin strips.
3. Mix the green chili paste, garlic paste and grated coconut pulp together and then grind them into a thick paste. This is the Masala paste.
4. Heat the cooking oil in a pan.
5. Once the oil is hot, add the onions followed by the boiled green peas and the masala paste. Stir for a minute and then add the beaten fresh Eggs to the pan.
6. Sprinkle corianders leaves into the pan and keep stirring slowly till the fresh Eggs are cooked.

Egg-Lemon Sauce

Ingredients:

2 cups Meat Broth

1 tsp Fennel seeds powder

Salt to taste

4 Fresh Eggs

4 tbsp fresh Lemon Juice

Instructions:

1. Separate the egg white from the fresh Eggs and beat it thoroughly.
2. Then add the yolks back and beat it again.
3. Add the fresh lemon juice, meat broth and fennel seed powder to the fresh Eggs .
4. Stir well and serve as a side dish and dip.

Egg-Tomato Curry

Ingredients:

1/2 tsp Garam Masala

2 Cloves

1 cm long Cinnamon Stick

Salt to taste

2 -2 tbsp Cooking Oil

4 Fresh Eggs

4 tbsp grated Coconut pulp

2 medium sized Tomato

2 medium sized Onion

2 tbsp fresh Coriander leaves

Instructions:

1. Hard boil the fresh Eggs , remove the cover and keep them aside.
2. Finely dice the Onion and tomato.
3. Heat the cooking oil in a pan.
4. Once the oil is hot, add the diced onion and tomato to the pan followed by the cloves and cinnamon stick.
5. Stir for a minute and then add grated coconut pulp, Garam masala and coriander leaves to the onion-tomato mixture and stir for a minute more.
6. Then add 5-7 cups of fresh water to the pan, cover with a lid and let it cook over medium heat for 6-8 minutes.
7. Once the curry is cooked, cut the fresh Eggs into 2 or 4 parts each and put them into the curry.
8. Now stir it slowly for 2-4 minutes more and serve hot.

Tomato Chicken

Ingredients:

2 tsp Garam Masala

2 tbsp Onion paste

2 Cups Tomato Puree

2 tbsp chopped Coriander leaves

2 tbsp grated Coconut pulp

Salt to taste

2 -2 tbsp Cooking Oil

250 gm Chicken (cut into small bite-sized pieces)

2 tbsp Lemon juice

1/2 tsp Turmeric Powder

1/2 tsp Cardamom Powder

1/2 tsp Clove Powder

Instructions:

1. Rub the lemon juice, turmeric powder, cardamom powder, clove powder to the Chicken pieces thoroughly and set it aside for 40-6 0 minutes.
2. Heat the cooking oil in a pan.
3. Once the oil is hot, add the onion paste and stir for a minute.
4. Then add tomato puree and Garam masala to the pan and stir for a couple of minutes.
5. Put the pieces of chicken in the pan, add salt to taste and stir slowly for 2-4 minutes.
6. Then cover the pan with a lid and let the chicken cook on medium heat.
7. Turn off the heat when the chicken is perfectly cooked. Garnish with fresh coriander leaves and grated coconut pulp and serve hot.

Boiled Chicken In Pink Stew

Ingredients:

2 cup fresh Beet (finely diced)

1/2 tsp Garam Masala

5-7 whole black Peppercorns

Salt to taste

1 tbsp Cooking Oil

2 6 0 gm Chicken (Chicken breasts cut into small bite sized pieces)

2 medium sized Onion (finely diced)

2 cups fresh Carrots (finely diced)

Instructions:
1. Heat the cooking oil in a large pot.
2. Once the oil is hot add onion, carrots and beet to the pot and stir for a minute.

3. Then add salt and Garam Masala and stir for a couple of minutes more on a medium heat.
4. Then add the chicken pieces followed by water. (pour in water till it covers the chicken pieces completely)
5. Then add the peppercorns to the pot and cover the pot with a lid.
6. Once the chicken is cooked, remove the lid and let the excess water evaporate a bit.
7. Garnish with fresh coriander leaves and serve hot.

Chicken In Coriander-Spinach Stew

Ingredients:

2 tbsp Tomato Puree

2 tbsp Fresh Lemon Juice

1/2 tsp Turmeric powder

1/2 tsp Garam Masala

Salt to taste

2-4 tbsp Cooking Oil

2 6 0 gm Chicken (Chicken breasts cut into small bite sized pieces)

2 cup fresh Coriander leaves (finely chopped)

4 cups fresh Spinach leaves

2 medium sized Onion (finely diced)

2 medium Potato (finely diced)

Instructions:

1. Heat the cooking oil in a pan.
2. Once the oil is hot, add spinach leaves and chopped coriander leaves and stir well till the spinach leaves wilt. (set the leaves aside in a bowl)
3. Heat the cooking oil in a pan.
4. Once the oil is hot, add the diced onion to the pan and stir till the onion turns brown.
5. Then add the chicken pieces and stir till the chicken turns light brown.
6. Then add diced potato, tomato puree, garam masala, turmeric powder, spinach-coriander leaves and salt.
7. Stir for a couple of minutes and add 4 cups of water to the pan.
8. Cover the pan with a lid and let the chicken cook over a medium heat.

9. Once the chicken is cooked, add the lemon juice and cook for a few minutes more before serving.

Mushroom Infused Grilled Chicken

Ingredients:

1 cup Chicken broth

1/2 tsp Garam Masala

2 tbsp Rice flour

Salt to taste

2 -2 tbsp Cooking Oil

2 6 0 gm Chicken (Chicken breasts cut into small bite sized pieces)

2-4 tbsp Lemon Juice

2 cup fresh Mushrooms (cut into thin slices)

Instructions:

1. Put the chicken breasts on a skewer, brush lemon juice onto the chicken pieces followed some small amount of Ghee (clarified butter) and then put them on a grill to cook.
2. Meanwhile, heat the cooking oil in a pan.
3. Once the oil is hot, add the sliced mushrooms to the pan and stir for a minute and then add the garam masala.
4. Keep stirring till the mushrooms turn brown and lose their excess moisture.
5. Then sprinkle the rice flour slowly on the mushrooms, all the while stirring continuously and keep stirring for a couple of minutes more.
6. Then add the chicken broth and salt to the pan and bring it to a boil.

7. Let it reduce to half, over medium heat.
8. While serving pour the mushroom mixture over the grilled chicken pieces.
9. Garnish with fresh coriander leaves and serve hot.

Green Pomfrets

Ingredients:

1/2 tsp Black Pepper Powder

2 tsp Tamarind Pulp

2 tsp Rice Flour

Salt to taste

2-4 tbsp Cooking Oil

2 medium sized Pomfret fish

2 tsp Ginger-Garlic Paste

2 tsp green Chili Paste

2 tsp paste of Coriander Leaves

Instructions:

1. Cut off the fins and tails of the fish. Remove the eyes.
2. Clean the fish and cut open its stomach and then wash it thoroughly.
3. Now slide in a knife and slit the fish open, length-wise to remove the central bone and then cut the fish into small bite-sized pieces.
4. Mix ginger-garlic paste, chili paste, coriander leaves paste, tamarind pulp and black pepper powder together and then rub this mixture to the pieces of Pomfrets and leave for 2 6 -25 minutes.
5. Then add rice flour to the pieces and mix it well.
6. Heat the cooking oil in a pan.
7. Once the oil is hot, shallow fry the pieces of fish in the pan. Flip it when

one side is cooked to cook the other side.
8. When the fish is almost cooked, spray a few drops of water on the fish and cover the pan with a lid and keep the lid on for a couple of minutes.
9. Garnish with fresh rings of onion and a slice of lemon. Serve hot.

Carrot Coconut Muffins

Ingredients

- 1 cup of coconut oil
- 2 teaspoon of vanilla extract
- 1/2 cup of any sweetener
- 2 teaspoons of ground cinnamon

- 1/2 cup of coconut flour
- 2 teaspoon of baking powder
- 2 cups of shredded carrots
- 2 large fresh Eggs

Instructions

1. Preheat oven to 450F. Line a 25 muffin tin with paper liners.
2. In a bowl, combine the coconut flour. Baking powder. Sweetener, cinnamon.
3. Add vanilla, sweetener, coconut oil, carrots and fresh Eggs to food processor. Blend until combined. Pour into dry

ingredients. Stir until combined. (Don't overmix.)
4. Pour batter in each tin to ⅔ full.
5. Bake 4 10 minutes.
6. Allow to cool 4 0 minutes. Serve.

Pumpkin Ice-Cream

Ingredients

- 1 teaspoon of nutmeg
- 21 teaspoons of ground cinnamon
- 1 teaspoon of ground ginger
- Pinch of salt
- 2 Tablespoon of gelatin

- 2 can of coconut milk
- 2 cup of unsweetened almond milk
- 2 cup of canned or fresh pumpkin puree
- 2 teaspoon of pure vanilla extract

Instructions

1. Dissolve gelatin in 1/2 cup boiling water.
2. Add rest of ingredients, including gelatin, to food processor. Blend until smooth.
3. Transfer mixture to a freezer-safe container. Cover. Freeze for 2 hours.
4. After 2 hours, use a wooden spoon to stir the ice-cream, to prevent crystalizing.
5. Leave in freezer overnight. Serve the following day.

Strawberry Gateau

Ingredients

- 4 large egg yolks
- 2 Tablespoons of butter
- 2 Tablespoons of coconut oil
- 1/2 cup of coconut flour
- 2 Tablespoons of heavy cream
- 1/2 cup of strawberries
- 1/2 teaspoon of baking powder
- 2 teaspoons of lemon juice
- Zest from 2 lemon
- 2 Tablespoons of any granulated sweetener
- 30 drops of any liquid sweetener

Instructions

1. Preheat oven to 450F. Line an 8x8 baking dish with parchment paper.
2. In a small bowl, combine the egg yolks.

3. Using a handheld mixer, whisk until pale and fluffy.
4. Add liquid sweetener and granulated sweetener. Whisk until fully combined.
5. Add heavy cream, butter, coconut oil, lemon juice, lemon zest. Whisk until smooth.
6. Add baking soda and coconut flour. Continue to whisk until combined.
7. Add the strawberries. Stir gently.
8. Transfer batter to baking dish. Bake 30 minutes.
9. Allow to cool 4 0 minutes before slicing. Serve.

Beetroot And Mustard Chips

Ingredients

- 2 Tablespoons of olive oil
- 2 pinches of ground mustard seeds
- 6 beets
- **Salt and pepper**

Instructions

1. Preheat oven to 450F. Grease 2 baking sheets with olive oil.
2. Peel and slice the beets thinly using a mandolin, or the wide angle on a (cheese) grater. Place beets in a bowl.
3. Toss with olive oil. Season with mustard seeds, salt and pepper.
4. Arrange beets in single layer on baking sheets. Bake 40 minutes, or become crispy.
5. Cool 6 minutes before serving.

Roasted Kale Chips

Ingredients

- 4 cups of chopped kale, throw away the stems
- 2 Tablespoons of extra virgin olive oil
- **Salt and pepper**

Instructions

1. Preheat the oven to 450F. Line a baking tray with parchment paper.
2. Place the kale in a large bowl. Drizzle with olive oil. Season with salt and pepper.
3. Arrange the kale in single layer on baking tray.
4. Bake 25 minutes, until they become crispy.
5. Serve hot or cold.

Parmesan Chips

Ingredients

- 1/2 cup of grated Parmesan
- Pinch of fresh ground pepper
- 1/2 cup of shaved Parmesan

Instructions

1. Preheat the oven to 450F. Line 2 baking trays with parchment paper.
2. In a small bowl, combine the two cheeses and pepper. Stir well.
3. Using a teaspoon, spoon mixture on baking tray. Pat it down until almost flat. Leave about 2 -2 inches space between piles. Repeat until you use all the mixture.
4. Bake in oven until golden brown and crispy, approximately 8 minutes.

5. Remove the baking tray from oven. Cool for 6 minutes before serving.

Devilled Fresh Eggs

Ingredients

- 4 Tablespoons of mayo
- 2 Tablespoon of Dijon mustard
- Splash of hot sauce
- 30 large fresh Eggs
- Paprika seasoning

Instructions

1. Place the fresh Eggs in a large pot. Fill pot with water until fresh Eggs are covered.
2. Boil 30 minutes.
3. Once cooked, rinse under cold water. Peel and rinse in cold water.

4. Cut the fresh Eggs in half. Remove the yolks. Yolks in one bowl, whites on a plate.
5. Add hot sauce, mayo to egg yolks. Mash yolks with a fork. Stir until combined.
6. Spoon the yolk filling into hollowed egg whites, or fill a Ziploc baggie, cut a corner off, not too wide, and fill the fresh Eggs , with a bump of egg yolk mixture above the white (as seen in picture).
7. Garnish with paprika seasoning. Refrigerate until ready to eat.

Cheesy Zucchini And Broccoli Soup

Ingredients

- 4 Tablespoons of virgin olive oil
- 6 cups of water
- Salt and pepper
- Parmesan cheese

- 4 large green zucchinis
- 2 cup of broccoli, cut into small pieces
- 2 leeks (the white part)

Instructions

1. In a large saucepan, heat the olive oil over medium heat. Add the leeks.
2. Cook until they are soft, stirring occasionally, approximately 30 minutes.
3. Add chopped broccoli and zucchinis. Sauté 10 minutes.

4. Add water. Simmer uncovered 30 minutes.
5. Using a handheld blender, blend the soup in the pot until smooth.
6. Transfer to bowls, sprinkle with cheese and serve.

Garlic Castilian Soup

Ingredients

- 4 cups of water
- 6 large fresh Eggs
- 2 thinly sliced red bell pepper
- 4 large cloves of garlic
- 2 Tablespoons of olive oil
- 4 cups of vegetable broth
- **Salt and pepper**

Instructions

1. Heat the oil over medium heat in a large saucepan. Sauté the garlic 4 minutes.
2. Add 2 cup of vegetable broth. Cover and simmer 30 minutes.
3. Using a fork, mash the garlic into a paste.
4. Pour in water and rest of vegetable broth. Bring to a boil. Add the red pepper.

Simmer 30 minutes. Break the fresh Eggs into the boiling soup.
5. Cook until the whites are solid, approximately 4 minutes. Serve immediately.

Dill And Leek Soup

Ingredients

- 2 cups of homemade vegetable broth
- 2 cups of water
- ¾ cup of heavy cream
- 2 Tablespoons of olive oil
- 2 Tablespoon of fresh dill, chopped
- 2 large green onions, chopped
- 2 large leeks
- 2 zucchini
- **Salt and pepper**

Instructions

1. Wash the leeks. Remove dark green leaves. (Keep some dark leaves for garnish.)
2. Grate the green part of the zucchini.

3. Place the zucchini, green onions, leeks, water, and vegetable broth in a deep pot. Cover and simmer 25 minutes.
4. Allow to cool for 30 minutes. Pour ingredients in a blender. Blend for a few seconds.
5. Return the mixture to a pot. Stir in the heavy cream. Season with salt and pepper.
6. Spoon into bowls. Garnish with dark leaves from leeks. Serve.

Grain-Free Vegan Mushroom Creamy Soup

Ingredients

- 1 teaspoon of extra virgin olive oil
- 2 1 cups of white button mushrooms, diced
- 1 yellow onion, diced
- Green onion for garnish, chopped
- 2 cups of cauliflower florets
- 2 1 cups of original almond milk unsweetened
- 2 teaspoon of onion powder
- 1/2 teaspoon of Himalayan rock salt
- Ground black pepper

Instructions

1. In a medium saucepan, combine almond milk, cauliflower, salt, pepper and onion powder. Cover and simmer on medium heat 8 minutes, until cauliflower is tender.
2. Allow to cool for 6 minutes before pouring into food processor.
3. Transfer to food processor.
4. Blend until smooth.
5. In a medium saucepan, heat some oil over medium heat.
6. Sauté onions and mushrooms until they soften, approximately 6-8 minutes.
7. Pour cauliflower mixture in with onions and mushrooms.
8. Cover and simmer 30 minutes. Soup will thicken.
9. Garnish with fresh green onion. Serve while hot.

Vegan Gazpacho

Ingredients

- 2 clove of garlic, minced
- 4 1 cups of tomato juice
- 1/2 cup of extra virgin olive oil
- 1/2 cup of white wine vinegar
- 1/2 cup of fresh parsley, finely chopped
- ⅛ teaspoon of powdered white stevia
- Salt and pepper
- 2 batch of croutons

- 2 medium red onion, finely chopped
- 4 medium tomatoes, finely chopped
- 1 medium cucumber, finely chopped
- 1 green pepper, de-seeded, finely chopped
- 6 celery stalks, finely chopped celery stalks

Instructions

1. Place all the ingredients in a large bowl. Stir together. Refrigerate 4 hours.
2. Serve in bowls. Garnish with croutons and fresh parsley.

Vegan Creamy Broccoli Soup

Ingredients

- 2 medium cauliflower, diced into florets
- 4 cups of unsweetened almond milk
- 4 cups broccoli florets
- 2 Tablespoon of onion powder

- 2 Tablespoon of extra virgin olive oil
- 2 yellow onion, sliced
- 2 teaspoon of sea salt
- Ground black pepper

Instructions

1. In a large saucepan, heat the oil over medium heat. Sauté onions 10 minutes.
2. Add a few tablespoons of water while frying to make sure it doesn't burn.
3. Add milk and cauliflower. Season with salt and pepper.
4. Cover and simmer 30 minutes.

5. Add half the broccoli.
6. Cook 30 minutes. Allow to cool slightly before placing in food processor.
7. Transfer ingredients to food processor. Blend until smooth.
8. Pour ingredients in saucepan.
9. Add onion powder and rest of the broccoli.
10. Cover and cook 30 minutes, soup will thicken up. Spoon into bowls. Serve while hot.

Mixed Greens Creamy Soup

Ingredients

- 1/2 cup of gluten-free vegetable broth
- 2 clove of garlic, minced
- 2 Tablespoon of soy seasoning
- 2 Tablespoon of lemon juice
- 2 pinch of chilli powder
- 2 cups of spinach leaves
- 2 avocado
- 1 cucumber
- 2 large green onion, chopped
- 1 cup of red bell peppers, chopped
- Ground black pepper

Instructions

1. Transfer ingredients listed to a food processor.
2. Blend 6 minutes, until smooth.
3. Pour into a medium saucepan.

4. Cover and simmer 10 minutes. Serve in bowls.

Tomato Soup

Ingredients

- 2 teaspoon of sea salt
- 1/2 cup of fresh basil
- 1 teaspoon of black pepper
- 2 clove of garlic
- 4 roma tomatoes
- 1 cup of sun dried tomatoes
- 1 cup of raw macadamia nuts
- 4 cups of hot water

Instructions

1. Transfer ingredients listed to food processor.
2. Blend 6 minutes, until smooth.
3. Pour into a medium saucepan.
4. Cover and simmer 10 minutes. Serve in bowls.

Wholly Appetizing Mango Chia Seed Pudding

Ingredients:

- 2 whole cup of 30 0ml coconut milk
- 4 tablespoon of chia seed
- 2 whole mango completely peeled up and pureed

Preparation:

1. This is a very straightforward recipe which only requires you to combine all of the mentioned ingredients in a bowl and let it chill for about an hour.

Chocolaty Cocoa Mousse

Ingredients:

- 4 tablespoon of cocoa
- 4 tablespoon of honey
- 2 teaspoon of vanilla extract
- Coconut cream scraped from the upper side of 25 4 .6 ounce chilled cans of full fat coconut milk

Preparation:

1. The first step is to open up your cans and scoop out the thick coconut cream and toss them to a large bowl

2. In that bowl, toss in the honey, cocoa, vanilla extract and beat using your mixer starting from low going all the way to medium until a nice foam appears

3. Divide the mixtures into even ramekins and chill them to your desired level of cold

Exquisite Pumpkin Nut Butter Cup

Ingredients:

- 1 a cup of organic pumpkin puree
- 1/2 teaspoon of organic ground nutmeg
- 1/2 teaspoon of organic ground ginger
- 2 teaspoon of organic ground cinnamon
- 2 /8 teaspoon of organic ground clove
- 2 teaspoon of organic vanilla extract
- 2 /2a cup of homemade almond butter
- 2 tablespoon of organic maple syrup
- 4 tablespoon of organic coconut oil

For Topping

- 4 tablespoon of organic maple syrup
- 2 cup of organic coconut oil
- 2 cup of organic raw cacao powder

Preparation:

1. Firstly you are going to need to make the pumpkin filling, to do this take a medium sized bowl and pour in all of the ingredients listed under pumpkin filling and mix them until creamy

2. For the chocolate topping, take another bowl and mix in all of the ingredients listed under chocolate topping until smooth and creamy

3. Then, take a muffin cup and fill about 2/4 of it with chocolate topping

4. Keep in freezer and chill for 30 minutes

5. Fill another 2/4 with pumpkin filling

6. And finally fill the last part with another layer of chocolate mix

7. Put in freezer and chill for 2 hours

Tender Chocolate Silk Pie

Ingredients:

- 2 and a 1 cup of cocoa powder
- 2 cup of heavy cream
- 2 tablespoon of vanilla
- 1 a teaspoon of espresso powder
- Just a pinch of salt

- 8 ounce of Dark Chocolate
- 1/2 cup of extra virgin olive oil
- 2 ripe Avocados
- 2 cup of coconut sugar

Preparation:

1. The first step here is to take a pan and toss in the dark chocolate in coconut oil at medium heat
2. Once done, let the chocolate cool at room temperature
3. Then scoop out some avocado meat and place them in a mixing bowl
4. Add the chocolate coconut mixture to the very bowl alongside cocoa powder and sugar
5. Whip up the mixture on medium speed using a mixer for about 2-4 minutes
6. Toss in the extract, cream, salt and espresso and whip it again on medium high to high speed for approximately 6 minutes until fully fluffy
7. Divide the batter into pie crust portions and chill them for a few hours.

Crunchy Cinnamon Apple Chips

Ingredients:

- 2 organic apples
- Cinnamon

Preparation:

The first step is to pre-heat your oven to a temperature of 250 degree Fahrenheit

Take a sharp knife and slice up your apples nicely

Line up a baking sheet using parchment paper and arrange the slices finely in a single layer

Lightly sprinkle some cinnamon over them

Bake for an hour and flip the slices over

Bake for another hour making sure that by the end, the slices are no longer moist

Turn your oven off and remove the chips allowing them to cool for about 30 minutes

Juice Popeye's Blueberry Smoothie

Ingredients:

- 1/2 cup of almond coconut milk
- 2 tablespoon of hemp hearts
- 2 tablespoon of vanilla whey protein powder
- 2 teaspoon of maca powder
- 2 teaspoon of maple syrup
- Bee pollen

- 1 of a frozen banana
- ¾ cup of frozen blueberries
- 2 handful of spinach leaves
- ¾ cup of nonfat honey Greek yogurt

Preparation:

1. No complicated step is required for this smoothie. Just toss in all of the ingredients into a blender and blend them at high

Palatable Candied Pecans

Ingredients:

- About 2 cups of pecans
- 2 whole egg white
- 2 tablespoon of water
- 1/2 cup of honey
- Pinch of sea salt
- Cinnamon as taste desires

Preparation:

1. Start off by pre-heating your oven to 30 0 degree Fahrenheit

2. In the mean time, take a bowl and toss in the egg white and water and whisk them nicely until frothy texture comes

3. Pour in the honey, cinnamon and salt and keep stirring it until all of the pecans are evenly coated

4. Spoon the pecans draining the liquid off them and place them into a parchment covered baking sheet

5. Spread out the pecans into a single fine layer
6. Bake for about 60 minutes stirring it for every 30 minutes
7. Spread them out on a glass cutting board to cool them down.

Crispy Balsamic Rosemary Roasted Vegetables

Ingredients:

- 2 chopped up zucchini chopped up into 2 inch chunks
- 1 of a red bell pepper chopped up into 2 inch pieces
- 2 minced up garlic clove
- 2 tablespoon of olive oil
- 2 tablespoon of balsamic vinegar
- 2 and a 1 tablespoon of fresh rosemary
- 1 a tablespoon of sea salt
- 1 a teaspoon of black pepper

- 2 cup of butternut squash chopped up into small cubes
- 2 and a 1 cup of broccoli florets chopped up into bite sized pieces
- 1 or a red onion chopped up into bite sized pieces

Preparation:

1. The first step here is to pre-heat your oven to 430 degree Fahrenheit
2. Mix up your vinegar, oil, pepper, salt in a large sized bowl
3. Toss in the vegetables and finely toss them to coat everything evenly
4. Spread out the mixture on a parchment paper lined up baking sheet.

Astonishingly Spiced And

Ingredients:

- 2 teaspoon of ground cumin
- 1 a teaspoon of smoked paprika
- Pinch of salt

- 4 cups of carrots sliced paper thin
- 2 tablespoon of olive oil

Preparation:

The first step here is to pre-heat your oven to a temperature of 230 degree Celsius

Slice up your carrot into paper thin shaped coins using a peeler if preferred

Place the slices in a bowl and toss them with the oil and spices to mix properly

Lay out the processed slices on a parchment paper lined baking sheet in a single layer and sprinkle some salt

Place it in the oven and let it bake for about 8-30 minutes making sure that they don't burn

Remove and serve hot!

Stunning Eggplant Caponata

Ingredients:

- 4 cups of chopped up tomatoes
- 4 tablespoon of white vinegar
- 2 tablespoon of capers
- 1 a cup of chopped up basil

- 2 tablespoon of olive oil
- 4 cloves of garlic
- 2 finely diced onion
- 4 cups of chopped up eggplant

Preparation:

1. Take a large frying pan and place it over medium heat and toss in the diced onions and garlic and cook for about 2-4 minutes

2. In the meantime, cut up the eggplants into approximately 1 inch sized cubes and toss them to the frying pan as well

3. Season it with salt
4. Cook the eggplant for about 6 minutes until it is soft and drizzle some olive oil on top
5. Toss in the chopped up tomatoes and vinegar to the pan and let the mixture finely simmer about 2 0-30 minutes until the tomatoes are tender.

Perfectly Sautéed Mushroom

Ingredients:

- 4 diced up garlic cloves
- 2 /4 cup of white win
- Salt as needed

- 2 tablespoon of butter
- 2 tablespoon of olive oil
- 2 and a 1 pound of gourmet mushroom

Preparation:

1. Take a heavy pan and heat it up
2. Pour in the oil and 1 of the butter
3. When almost smoking appeared, toss in the mushrooms
4. Keep stirring the mushroom until finely brown

5. Toss in another 1 butter and garlic
6. Stir everything quickly making sure to not burn it
7. Add in the white wine and let it cook

Sweetly Sautéed Radishes

Ingredients:

- 2 tablespoon of honey
- 2 tablespoon of white balsamic
- 1/2 teaspoon of sea salt
- 2 bunches of radishes about 25 in total
- 2 tablespoon of divided olive oil
- 2 teaspoon of butter
-

Preparation:

1. Start off by Sauté the radishes and gently keep them on the side

2. Prepare your glaze and pouring it into a oven proof dish and toss in the sautéed radishes, cover up the dish and keep it on the side

3. Set the radish greens and sliced radishes taking them in two separated bowls

4. 30 minutes you are in mood to serve, just pop the sautéed radishes into your oven at 4 6 0 degree Fahrenheit and keep them for until they are warm enough

5. Remove them from the oven and toss in the radish greens to the dish and keep tossing until finely wilt

Gracefully Roasted Heirloom Carrots

Ingredients:

- 1 a tablespoon of coconut oil
- 2 tablespoon of maple syrup
- 2 /8 cup of fresh squeeze orange juices
- 2 /8 teaspoon of sea salt
- Salt as needed

- 2 bunch of fine heirloom carrots
- 2 tablespoon of fresh thyme leaves

Preparation:

Start of by preheating your oven to 4 6 0 degree Fahrenheit

Thoroughly wash up dry carrots and remove any green parts

Take a small mixing bowl and combine the coconut oil alongside the maple syrup, orange juice and sea salt

Pour over your carrots and spread them evenly on a large baking sheet

Sprinkle it with thyme and roast for about 46 minutes

Intensely Blistered Beans With Crushed Almond

Ingredients:

- 2 and a 1 tablespoon of minced up fresh dill
- Juice of just one lemon
- 1/2 cup of crushed up almonds
- Flaky sea salt for finishing
- 2 pound of fresh green beans with their ends trimmed up
- 2 and a 1 tablespoon of olive oil
- 1/2 teaspoon of salt

Preparation:

1. Start off by pre-heating your oven to 400 degree Fahrenheit
2. Toss in the green beans with your olive oil and also with salt

3. Then spread them in one single layer on a large sized sheet pan
4. Roast it up for 30 minutes and stir it nicely, then roast for another 8-30 minutes
5. Remove it from the oven and keep stirring in the lemon juice alongside the dill

Perplexing Cauliflower Couscous With Apricots And

Ingredients:

- 4 tablespoon of chopped up parsley
- 2 tablespoon of chopped up cilantro
- 1/2 teaspoon of red pepper flakes
- Salt as needed
- Pepper as needed

- 2 heads up cauliflower
- 1 a cup of roasted cashew nut
- 2 /4 cup of apricots cut up into raisin sized pieces
- 4 finely chopped up scallions
  For the Dressing

- 2 tablespoon of fresh lemon juice
- 2 tablespoon of orange juice
- 2 teaspoon of grated fresh ginger
- 1 a teaspoon of ground cinnamon
- Salt as needed

- Pepper as needed
- 2 tablespoon of dates
- 2 tablespoon of olive oil
- 2 tablespoon of water

Preparation:

1. The first step is to pre-heat your oven to 430 degree Fahrenheit
2. Gently make the cauliflower couscous and coarsely chop up your cauliflower into florets and toss in your food processor
3. Process them until a fine texture and consistency has appeared
4. Spread out the cauliflower couscous evenly on a baking dish and bake for about 2 6 -25 minutes, keep stirring everything halfway through
5. Gently remove it from oven once done and let it cool

6. For the dressing, toss in all of the ingredients into a high speed blender and blend until a fine and smooth, creamy texture has been achieved
7. Once the cauliflower couscous has been cooled up, take a large sized mixing bowl and stir in the dressing gently

Spring Chicken Salad

Ingredients:

1 cup shallots, chopped

2 tbsp parsley, chopped

2 tbsp olive oil

2 tbsp lime juice

2 tsp garlic powder

Sea salt and pepper

2 chicken breasts, baked and cut into bite-sized pieces

2 avocado, cubed

2 cup apple, cubed

1/2 cup celery, chopped

Directions:

1. Blend together the olive oil, lime juice, garlic powder, parsley, salt and pepper to a fine dressing.
2. In a salad bowl, toss in the remaining ingredients.
3. Drizzle the dressing over the salad.
4. Coat the dressing all over the salad, by gently flipping the bowl. Serve.

Raw Kale Salad

Ingredients:

1/2 cup walnuts, minced

1 cup almonds, sliced

1 cup pomegranates

2 tbsp cilantro, chopped

4 cups fresh kale

2 cup strawberries

4 carrots, grated

Dressing:

2 cup olive oil

Sea salt and pepper

2 cup red wine vinegar

2 tsp garlic powder

2 tsp mint leaves, chopped

2 tsp mustard

Directions:

1. Wash the kale. Pat dry. Lay the leaves in a salad bowl and add in all the remaining ingredients.
2. In a separate bowl, beat all the ingredients for the dressing. Whip straight away prior to serving to make sure that the olive oil and vinegar have not split.
3. Pour the dressing on the salad. Toss and serve.

Creamed Spinach

Ingredients:

1/2 tsp ground nutmeg

2 tsp chili powder

2 tbsp cornstarch

4 tbsp ghee

Sea salt and pepper

4 cups spinach

2 onion, chopped

4 garlic cloves, crushed

2 cups coconut milk

Directions:

1. Heat a skillet on a medium heat. Add ghee. Ghee should not brown, so avoid extreme temperatures.
2. Mix the cornstarch with some warm water. Slowly pour the mixture into the dissolved ghee.
3. Toss in the onion and garlic. Cook till transparent.
4. Add all the spinach. Boil until the leaves are tender.
5. Pour in the coconut milk, nutmeg, and chili powder. Stir well. Simmer till the dish is creamy.
6. Season to taste with salt and pepper.
7. If the sauce is not sufficiently creamy, whisk a teaspoon of cornstarch with some coconut milk and gradually pour this mixture into the spinach. Make sure to let it simmer for a minute or two.
8. Serve.

Roasted Thyme Mushroom

Ingredients:

6 thyme sprigs

4 tbsp olive oil

Ghee
Sea salt and pepper

2 cup mushrooms of your choice

4 garlic cloves, crushed

Directions:

1. Preheat the oven to 490 ºF.
2. Spread ghee, garlic, and thyme sprigs on a baking tray.
3. Arrange the mushrooms with the cap side facing the tray, over the thyme and garlic.

4. Sprinkle the mushrooms with salt and pepper.
5. Douse with the olive oil. Roast in the oven for 30 minutes.
6. Remove the baking tray from oven. Drizzle the mushrooms with the juice that remains.

Creamy Chicken Onion Soup

Ingredients:

4 cups stock of your choice

2 cup full fat coconut milk

2 tbsp cilantro, minced

Grass-fed cow's butter

Sea salt and pepper

2 cup red onion, chopped

2 cups chicken, baked and diced

2 tsp garlic powder

2 tbsp cornstarch

Directions:

1. Heat a skillet on a medium heat. Add ghee to it.
2. After the ghee is fully dissolved, add the onions to the saucepan. Cook until transparent.
3. Slowly pour in the chicken stock. Bring to a gentle simmer.
4. Add the chicken and coconut milk while stirring continuously.
5. Lower the heat. Let cook till the chicken has absorbed all the flavors and doubles in size, for about 30 minutes.
6. Ladle about 1 a cup of the soup and in a small bowl, mix with the cornstarch, till there are no lumps. Gradually pour this mixture into the soup, while stirring steadily, till creating the desired consistency.

7. Season with salt and pepper. Sprinkle the cilantro on top before serving. Serve warm.

Grand Pumpkin Soup

Ingredients:

2 cup spring onions, minced

4 cups stock of your choice

4 cups pumpkin, chopped

2 cup coconut cream

Sea salt and pepper

1 cup bell pepper, cubed

4 cloves garlic, minced

2 tsp ground cumin

2 tbsp coconut oil

Directions:

1. Stir fry the onions with the coconut oil in a sauce pan over a medium heat for few minutes.
2. Stir often to avoid burning the onions.
3. Add the garlic and bell peppers to the pan.
4. Cook for just about 6 minutes to allow the vegetables to soften.
5. Add in the cumin.
6. Stir well.
7. Pour in the stock and the pumpkin.
8. Bring to a simmer.
9. Let it cook for around 30 minutes, or until the pumpkin is tender and breaks easily.
10. Take out the soup from the stove. Mix in the coconut cream, little by little.
11. Add salt and pepper to taste.
12. When cooled, use a blender to purée the soup and serve warm.

Mushroom Mussels Chowder

Ingredients:

4 bacon slices

1 cup cucumber, chopped

4 garlic cloves, minced

2 tbsp chili powder

2 cups coconut milk

Fresh parsley, chopped

Sea salt and pepper

2 lbs mussels, washed

2 cup button mushrooms, color of your choice

2 cup sweet potatoes, cubed

2 cup leeks, chopped

2 red onion, sliced

Directions:

1. In a large saucepan, bring 4 cups of water to the boil.
2. Add the sweet potatoes into the boiling water for 10 minutes. Carefully, with the help of a slotted spoon, remove the sweet potatoes and set aside, but keep the water in the pan.
3. In a separate pan, cook the bacon, frequently turning over for about 10 minutes.
4. Add the onion, garlic, mushrooms, leeks, and cucumber. Cook for another 4 minutes.
5. Add the boiled sweet potatoes and chili powder. Stir well.
6. Add sea salt and pepper to taste.
7. Pour in the coconut milk and fold.
8. Pour in a cup of the water in which you boiled the potatoes. Mix again.

9. Bring to a simmer and drop in the mussels.
10. Cover the pan and cook for ten minutes.
11. Serve with fresh parsley sprinkled on top.

The Best Vegetable Soup

Ingredients:

2 garlic cloves, crushed

2 tsp cumin powder

2 stick of cinnamon

6 cups vegetable stock

2 tbsp parsley, chopped

Sea salt and pepper

2 cups kale, chopped

2 cups cabbage, chopped

1/2 cup shallots, chopped

2 celery stalks, chopped

4 carrots, minced

2 tbsp ghee

2 cup cauliflower, in florets

2 cup cherry tomatoes, quartered

2 tbsp ginger, grated

Directions:

1. In a pot, add ghee. When it melts, add the onion, cinnamon, ginger, and garlic over a medium heat.
2. Cook for 2 to 4 minutes, mixing well, until fragrant.
3. Add the celery, carrots, and tomatoes.
4. Stir the whole thing to mix, and cook till tender.

5. Stir in the cumin and salt and pepper to taste.
6. Add in the cauliflower, cabbage, and vegetable stock, and bring to a simmer.
7. Decrease the heat and cook for around 30 minutes.
8. Finally, toss in the kale a few minutes before serving. Serve hot.

Turkey Potage

Ingredients:

2 cup cauliflower, boiled and shredded

2 cup cabbage, cut into strips

2 bay leaves

2 garlic cloves, crushed

2 rosemary sprigs

2 tsp thyme

Sea salt and pepper

2 cups turkey, cooked and chopped

2 leek, chopped

4 carrots, chopped

2 cup bell peppers, diced

2 celery stalks, chopped

Turkey Stock:

6 garlic cloves, halved

4 thyme sprigs

2 bay leaf

1 tsp cumin powder

4 cups cold water

4 lbs turkey parts, preferably bones

2 onions, chopped

2 celery ribs, cut into chunks

2 carrots, quartered

Pepper

Directions:

1. Lay the turkey parts in a crockpot, and toss in all of the turkey stock ingredients.
2. Season generously with pepper.
3. Fill the pot with water and let it boil.
4. Lower heat to a light boil, and cook for 4 to 8 hours.
5. Drain the stock with a sieve, discarding all the remaining ingredients. Set aside the stock, letting it cool.
6. Put in all the components for the soup in a larger pot.
7. Fill up the pan with the turkey stock, and season to taste.
8. Bring to a boil, and let it cook for 410 minutes.

Grandma's Apple Ketchup

Ingredients:

2 bell pepper, diced

2 cup raw apple cider vinegar

2 cup raw honey

25 red tomatoes, skinned and chopped

6 apples, peeled, cored, and chopped

2 pear, peeled, cored, and minced

2 onions, chopped

Pickling Spices:

1/2 tsp ground ginger

1 tsp red pepper flakes

2 bay leaf, crushed

2 cinnamon stick

2 tbsp mustard seed

2 tsp allspice

2 tsp coriander seeds

2 clove

Sea salt

Directions:

1. Lay the pickling spices ingredients in cheesecloth and tie it tightly like a closed bundle.

2. Mix all the ingredients, including the spice bundle, in a large pot and set over a medium heat.
3. Bring the ketchup to a simmer, stirring regularly.
4. Lower the temperature to the lowest setting and let cook for 2 hour, uncovered, stirring sporadically.
5. Remove the spice bundle.
6. Pour into warm, sterilized jars.
7. Let chill and keep cold.

Coconut Mayonnaise

Ingredients:

4 tsp lemon juice

1 cup olive oil

1 cup coconut oil

2 egg yolks

1 tsp mustard

Directions:

1. In a bowl, beat the yolks, mustard, and 2 tsp lemon juice, using a food processor or blender.
2. Start whisking briskly, with the blender speed on low, while trickling the oil at a snail's pace, even drop by drop at the start. Since you are creating a perfect emulsion, take your time trickling the oil, as pouring it too fast can completely wreck the dish.
3. Beat without a break.
4. As you add more oil, the blend will form and the mayonnaise will start to condense

and you can tip the oil more rapidly at this point.
5. When all the oil is included and the mayonnaise is substantial, beat in the rest of the lemon juice.
6. Season with salt and pepper.
7. Keep chilled at all times.

Paleo Salsa Verde

Ingredients:

1 cup cilantro, minced

2 tbsp lime juice

2 jalapeño pepper, chopped

1 cup red onion, chopped

2 lb green tomatillos, de-husked

Salt and pepper

Directions:

1. Halve the tomatillos lengthwise and sear them either on the grill or using a broiler until the skin has darkened considerably.
2. Put the seared tomatillos, onion, cilantro, lime juice, and jalapeño in a blender or food processor.
3. Blend into a silky pulp.
4. Place in the refrigerator to cool and serve at room temperature.

Sausage Casserole

Ingredients:

2 red onions, diced

⅓ cup almond milk

Ghee

Fresh cilantro, chopped

Sea salt and pepper

8 fresh Eggs

2 lb premium grass-fed sausage, without casing

2 sweet potatoes, medium-sized, chopped

2 green onion, sliced

2 bell pepper, diced

4 garlic cloves, crushed

Directions:

1. Preheat the oven to 490 ºF.
2. Melt some ghee in a pan over a medium-high temperature.
3. Toss in the sausages and crush while cooking.
4. When the sausages are no longer pink, transfer them to a spacious bowl.
5. Add the red onions, garlic, and bell pepper to the same pan. Cook over a medium heat till the vegetables are tender.
6. Transfer the vegetables into the bowl with the sausages.
7. Put the sweet potatoes in the pan, season with salt and pepper, and cook about 8 minutes, flipping them often to avoid uneven cooking.
8. When the sweet potatoes are softer, add them into the bowl with the sausages.
9. Scoop out the sausage and sweet potato mixture to a shallow oven-safe dish.

10. In a bowl, beat the fresh Eggs and almond milk, adding salt and pepper to taste.
11. Transfer the egg blend over the sausage mixture, and put in the oven.
12. Bake for 30 minutes, and serve warm, with green onions and cilantro sprinkled lavishly.

Tangy Herb Frittata

Ingredients:

4 cups baby spinach leaves

4 cherry tomatoes, sliced

4 tsp mustard

Fresh basil leaves, minced

2 tbsp coconut oil

Sea salt and pepper

25 fresh Eggs , large

6 bacon slices, diced

2 red onion, sliced

1 cup leeks, chopped

Directions:

1. Preheat the oven to 4 6 0ºF.
2. Beat the fresh Eggs and mustard in a bowl, and add salt and pepper to taste.
3. Heat the oil in an oven-safe pan over a medium heat.
4. Fry the bacon, onion and leeks until the onion is transparent.
5. Toss in the spinach to the pan and cook until the spinach withers.
6. Gradually pour the egg mixture into the skillet. Cook until it congeals just a bit. Arrange the tomatoes on top.
7. Just as the frittata is solid around the edges but still gooey in the center, move the pan to the oven and bake for 25 minutes till the frittata turns to a golden brown.
8. Top with basil leaves and serve warm.

Chicken Burrito

Ingredients:

2 red bell pepper, diced

1/2 tsp chili flakes

Coconut oil

6 whole-meal tortillas

Sea salt and pepper

6 fresh Eggs

2 chicken breast, thinly sliced

2 tomato, diced

1 onion, diced

Directions:

1. Heat the coconut oil in a pan over a medium-high heat.
2. Sauté the onion, bell pepper, and chili flakes until the onions are soft.
3. Add the tomato and cook for another minute or two.
4. In a separate bowl, beat the fresh Eggs and pour them over the cooking vegetables.
5. Using a fork, scramble the fresh Eggs until cooked throughout.
6. Pop a tortilla onto a skillet for a minute to soften, and then place onto a board.
7. Spoon some of the filling into the tortilla, then carefully roll and tuck in.
8. Repeat as directed for all the other tortillas.
9. Serve the burritos hot, with fresh salsa.

Salmon Cakes

Ingredients:

1 tsp garlic powder

2 tsp lime zest

2 egg, beaten

4 tbsp coconut oil

Fresh coriander leaves, minced

Sea salt and pepper

2 cups salmon, baked and flaked

2 sweet potatoes

2 onions, minced

2 tbsp fresh dill, minced

2 tbsp mustard

Directions:

1. Lay the sweet potatoes in a steep saucepan and fill up with cold water to cover by an inch.
2. Let the water boil over a medium heat. Lower the heat, cover, and let cook for 30 to 25 minutes.
3. Strain the water and rest the potatoes in a large bowl. Mash thoroughly with a fork and let cool.
4. When the potatoes are completely cooled, mix in the salmon, garlic powder, onion, dill, mustard, lime zest, egg, sea salt, and black pepper.
5. Gently stir everything until well integrated.
6. Shape the salmon mix into uniform patties.

7. Add the coconut oil in pan over a medium-high heat, and drop in the patties, cooking them for five minutes on each side.
8. Serve up the salmon cakes hot, with a sprinkling of coriander leaves.

Fish Tacos

Ingredients:

1 tsp garlic powder

2 jalapeño pepper, thinly chopped

2 cups tomatoes, diced

1 cup fresh cilantro, minced

4 tbsp lime juice

Sea salt and pepper

2 lb tilapia fillets

2 tbsp ghee

2 onion, diced

1 cup leeks, chopped

2 avocado, cubed

Directions:

1. In a big pan, heat the ghee on a medium heat. Add the leeks and onion.
2. Sauté the onions and leeks till the onions are transparent and the leeks fragrant.
3. Add the tilapia fillets to the pan.
4. Let the fillets cook for 6 minutes on each side before flipping to the other side. As the fish is cooking through, break it apart into flaky bits, with a fork.
5. Add the jalapeño pepper, tomatoes, cilantro, and lime juice to the blend. Season with salt and pepper.
6. Cook for 4 more minutes before removing from heat.

7. Serve the taco filling on a taco shell of your choice and top with avocado.

Lemon Lobster Salad

Ingredients:

1 cup zucchini, chopped

4 onion, finely chopped

4 tbsp lemon juice

Sea salt and pepper

Romaine lettuce leaves

4 lbs lobster tails

2 avocado, cubed

1 cup Paleo mayonnaise

Directions:

1. Fill up a large pot with water and a tablespoon of salt. Bring to a boil.
2. As the water is set to boil, organize an ice-water bath that will house all of the lobster tails immediately after boiling.
3. Drop the lobster tails into the boiling water. Boil for 30 minutes, until the shells take on a bright red hue.
4. Carefully take the tails from the boiling water and straight away transfer to the ice-water bath.
5. Let them sit for 2 minutes, then strain the water.
6. Halve the tails lengthwise to take out the meat from the shell.
7. Cut the lobster meat into bite sized bits, and gently pat dry with a paper towel and place in the refrigerator for 30 minutes to chill the lobster further.

8. In a larger bowl, mix the mayonnaise, onion, zucchini, and lemon juice, adding salt and pepper to taste.
9. Once the tails have been totally cooled, add them to the blend and gently fold to incorporate.
10. Place back in the refrigerator for another 30 minutes to allow the flavors to bond.
11. Serve the lobster salad chilled over romaine lettuce leaves and with avocado.

Tropical Chicken Fingers

Ingredients:

2 fresh Eggs

1/2 cup full-fat coconut milk

¾ cup coconut, shredded

Sea salt and pepper

2 chicken breasts, de-boned

1 cup coconut flour

Directions:

1. Preheat the oven to 400ºF.
2. With a heavy object, pound the chicken breasts so that they are leveled to an even width.
3. Cut the chicken into fingers that are around ¾ to 2 inch thick.
4. Beat the fresh Eggs and coconut milk together till slightly frothy.
5. Cover each chicken finger in the coconut flour, then submerge in the egg and coconut milk blend and lastly, douse in the shredded coconut.

6. When preparations for all the chicken fingers are done, assemble them on a large baking tray, and bake for 30 minutes, until chicken has been cooked throughout.
7. Serve hot with Grandma's Apple Ketchup.

Slow Cooker Rustic Chicken Chili

Ingredients:

2 cups salsa

2 tsp ground cumin

2 garlic cloves, minced

4 cups water

2 tsp chili powder

2 avocado, chopped

2 lb chicken breasts

4 bell peppers, cubed

2 red onion, minced

2 jalapeño pepper, chopped

Sea salt and pepper

Directions:

1. In a slow cooker, mix the chicken breasts, garlic, salsa, water, cumin, chili powder, and onion. Season with salt and pepper to taste.
2. Put on the lid. Cook on low for 6 to 8 hours.
3. Once it is done, take the chicken breasts up, and shred them with a fork, and return to the slow cooker.

4. Add the bell peppers and jalapeño in a large pan over a high heat and roast well.
5. Toss in the charred peppers and jalapeño to the slow cooker.
6. Give everything a good stir, and cover.
7. Let the chili cook for another 25 minutes. Add water to reach the preferred consistency, if needed.
8. Sprinkle avocado before serving. Serve hot.

Masala Chicken And Cauliflower Rice

Ingredients:

2 tsp curry powder

1 cup peas, parboiled

6 tbsp lemon juice

- 1 cup raw cashews
- 2 cup full-fat coconut milk
- 2 tbsp ginger, shredded
- 2 garlic cloves, crushed
- 2 tsp ground coriander
- 1 tsp ground cinnamon
- 1 tsp ground cumin
- 1 tsp red chili flakes
- 1/2 cup water
- 2 lb chicken breasts, cut into bite-sized pieces
- 2 head cauliflower, cut into florets
- 2 carrots, cubed
- 2 red bell pepper, diced
- 1 onion, chopped
- Ghee
- Sea salt and black pepper

Directions:

1. Heat a dry pan over a medium heat and lightly roast the cashew nuts until golden brown for about 2 minutes. Set aside to cool.
2. Put the cauliflower florets into a food processor. Pulsate until the cauliflower florets resemble a grain of rice. Do not over-blend the cauliflower or it may turn to pulp. I recommend you work in batches so you can keep an even consistency.
3. Once the florets are done, heat 2 tablespoons of ghee in a large frying pan over a medium heat.
4. Add the cauliflower and season with salt and pepper, folding to mix well.
5. Keep on cooking for another ten minutes, until the cauliflower is soft.
6. Transfer to a bowl, wrap to keep warm. Set aside.

7. Heat a large pan with 2 tablespoons of ghee over a medium heat.
8. Add the chicken, season with salt and pepper, cook for ten minutes, stirring sporadically, until the chicken is cooked throughout.
9. While the chicken is cooking, add the coconut milk, ginger, garlic cloves, curry powder, coriander, cinnamon, cumin, chili flakes and a handful of the roasted cashews into a blender or food processor.
10. Blend until a silky purée is formed.
11. Once the chicken is done, drop in the carrots, bell pepper, onion, and peas to the pan. Season with salt and pepper, and mix to combine well.
12. Let it simmer for a few minutes, and then pour in the lemon juice. Stir well and keep on cooking for 4 more minutes.
13. Add the purée and fold.
14. If the texture is very solid, add 1 cup of water to even it out.

15. Let the chicken and vegetables cook for 6 minutes, so that the new flavors can merge and meld.
16. Serve the masala chicken over cauliflower rice and sprinkle with roasted cashews.

Texan Bbq Meatballs

Ingredients:

1/2 cup almond flour

2 egg

1 tsp chili powder

1 tsp cumin powder

Coconut oil

Sea salt and pepper

2 lb ground beef

1 cup onions, sliced

BBQ sauce:

2 tbsp raw honey

2 tsp cornstarch

1 tsp chili powder

1 tsp cayenne pepper powder

1/2 tsp hot sauce

Sea salt and pepper

2 cup Paleo ketchup

2 onion, minced

2 tbsp raw apple cider vinegar

Directions:

1. Preheat the oven to 4 6 0ºF.
2. In a big bowl, mix the ground beef, onions, egg, almond flour, and chili powder. Season with salt and pepper. Mix well.
3. Roll the beef mixture into balls and set aside.
4. Heat some coconut oil in a shallow pan set over a medium heat. Fry the meatballs for

6 minutes on each side, then place them in a baking tray.
5. Mix all the ingredients for the BBQ sauce in a bowl. Season to taste. Stir until mixed.
6. Drizzle the sauce over the meatballs. Bake in the oven for 410 minutes.

'Guilt-Free' Taco Pie

Ingredients:

Pie Crust:

1 cup grass-fed cow's butter, melted

4 tsp salt

2 cups almond flour

Pie Filling:

- 2 cup spinach, chopped
- 2 bell pepper, cubed
- 2 avocado, diced
- 2 tsp rosemary, chopped
- Sea salt and pepper
- 2 lb ground beef
- 2 tbsp coconut oil
- 2 onion, chopped
- ¾ cup Paleo barbecue sauce (see recipe above)

Directions:

1. Combine almond flour, butter and salt in a large bowl. Mix with a fork, until a

crumbly texture takes shape, and gently knead to form a dough.
2. Transfer the dough into a 10-inch pie dish. Press it out uniformly into the dish so that the entire shell is covered.
3. Preheat the oven to 460ºF.
4. In a saucepan, over a medium-high heat, add the coconut oil, onion, and spinach. Brown the onions in the oil, until they become translucent and the spinach wilted.
5. Mix the ground beef to the cooked vegetables. Fry until the beef has cooked through.
6. Pour in the barbecue sauce with the beef. Season with salt and pepper.
7. Let the blend simmer for five more minutes. Remove from the heat. Stir in some rosemary.
8. Arrange the beef filling in the pie crust. Place in the oven for 410 minutes.
9. Before serving, garnish the surface of the pie with bell pepper and avocado.

Classic Coconut Tapioca Pudding

Ingredients:

2 vanilla bean

4 egg yolks

4 tbsp raw honey

1 cup tapioca pearls

4 cups full-fat coconut milk

Directions:

1. In a shallow-bottomed pan, mix the tapioca, 2 cups of coconut milk, and the vanilla bean over a medium heat.
2. Bring to a light boil over a moderate heat. Beat frequently, until the tapioca is clear and tender.
3. Gently pour in the remaining coconut milk.
4. Beat the egg yolks with the honey until smooth, in a small bowl.
5. Scoop out about half a cup of the hot coconut milk and very carefully and slowly drip it into the egg yolks while continuing to whisk them.
6. This should be done very carefully, as trickling the milk too fast will scramble the fresh Eggs .
7. After the egg mix is starting to froth, pour it back into the saucepan, stirring continuously.
8. Refrigerate the pudding until firm, and serve chilled.

Pumpkin Cookies

Ingredients:

1 cup coconut flour

1 tsp ground cinnamon

1/2 tsp ground ginger

1 tsp ground nutmeg

Sea salt

2 cups pumpkin purée

1 cup applesauce

1 cup coconut milk

2 tsp vanilla

2 cup almond meal

Directions:

1. Preheat the oven to 460ºF.
2. In a bowl, mix the pumpkin purée, salt, applesauce, coconut milk, and vanilla, until well combined.
3. Gradually add the coconut flour and almond meal, while folding the batter.
4. On a lightly greased baking tray, drop spoonfuls of the cookie mixture, and then compress with a fork.
5. Place the tray in the oven. Bake for 30 minutes.

Balsamic Cremini Roast Beef

Ingredients:

2 tbsp onion flakes

4 tbsp garlic flakes

1 tsp oregano, dried

1 tsp basil, dried

Sea salt and pepper

4 lbs beef rib roast

2 cups beef stock

1 cup cremini mushrooms, halved

1/2 cup balsamic vinegar

Directions:

1. Preheat the oven to 4 30 ºF.
2. In a bowl, combine the garlic, onion, oregano, salt, and pepper to make a mixture.
3. Rub the seasoning blend all over the roast, making sure that every inch is covered.
4. Place the roast on a rack in a roasting pan.
5. Roast in the preheated oven, uncovered, for 2 hours.
6. Remove the roast from the oven. Set aside for about 30 minutes.
7. While the meat is cooling, pour the beef stock into the pan, over a medium-high heat.
8. Pour in the vinegar.
9. Bring to a boil. Cook until reduced. Season to taste.
10. Drop in the mushrooms. Cook until they are soft.

11. Serve the rib roast with the balsamic-cremini sauce.

Coconut Milk Hot Chocolate

Ingredients:

1 cup dark chocolate, chopped

1/2 tsp vanilla extract

2 cups full-fat coconut milk

Directions:

1. Heat the coconut milk in a saucepan over a medium heat until hot. Do not let it boil.
2. Drop in the chocolate and vanilla extract. Stir until fully dissolved.
3. Serve hot.

Banana Pumpkin Booster

Ingredients:

1 cup almond milk

1 tsp ground cinnamon

1/2 tsp ground ginger

1 tsp ground nutmeg

2 cup pure pumpkin purée

4 bananas

Ice cubes

Directions:

1. Add the pumpkin purée, banana, almond milk, and the spices to a blender.
2. Blend until well incorporated.
3. Add the ice to the smoothie. Continue blending, until a silky texture forms.
4. Serve the booster cold.

Maple Date Brownies

Ingredients:

2 tbsp cocoa powder

1 cup organic peanut butter

4 tbsp maple syrup

4 tbsp almond milk

2 tbsp coconut oil

2 cups dates of your choice

1 cup hazelnuts, minced

4 tbsp almonds, minced

Sea salt

Directions:

1. Tenderize the dates by pounding with a rolling pin to soften them.
2. Blend the dates, hazelnuts, almonds, and cocoa powder, until it forms a thick consistency. Spread it on a greased baking tray.
3. Freeze the brownies for at least ten minutes.
4. Meanwhile, mix peanut butter, salt, maple syrup, almond milk, and coconut oil until creamy.
5. Spread the mixture on the brownies, cut into squares. Keep refrigerated.

Grilled Lemon Herb Lamb Chops

Ingredients:

4 tbsp garlic, minced

1/2 cup fresh lemon juice

1 cup olive oil

Sea salt and black pepper

6 lamb chops, thick-cut

1/2 cup basil leaves, minced

1/2 cup parsley, minced

4 tbsp scallions, minced

Directions:

1. Mix the basil, parsley, chives, garlic, lemon juice, and olive oil. Season with salt and pepper.
2. Pour the lemon-basil blend over the lamb chops and let marinate at room temperature for 4 0 minutes.
3. Preheat grill to medium-high heat.
4. Grill the lamb chops 4 to 6 minutes per side, depending on your preference.
5. Let the chops rest 6 minutes before serving.

Pacific Passion Steak

Ingredients:

1 cup beef stock

1/2 cup passion fruit purée

2 tbsp cumin

Olive oil

Sea salt and pepper

2 lbs sirloin tip steak, sliced

2 1 onions, minced

2 tomatoes, quartered

2 garlic cloves, crushed

Directions:

1. Spice up the steak with sea salt and pepper.
2. Add some olive oil in a pan over a medium-high heat.
3. Sear the steak for 10 minutes. Set aside.
4. Add more olive oil to the pan.
5. Lower the temperature to medium. Add the onions.
6. Cook till the onions are golden.
7. Add the garlic. Fry till fragrant.
8. Toss in the tomatoes.
9. Sprinkle sea salt and pepper.
10. Pour the beef stock into the pan. Simmer, stirring frequently, until tomatoes are tender.
11. Drop the steak back to the pan. Season with cumin. Pour the passion fruit purée into the mixture.
12. Let cook till the sauce is absorbed by the steak.

13. Serve hot.

Sour And Spicy Tuna

Ingredients:

2 garlic cloves, chopped

1/2 cup olive oil

4 tbsp lime juice

1 cup coriander, chopped

2 tbsp hot sauce

Sea salt and pepper

6 yellow fin tuna steaks

2 tsp cumin

1 tsp marjoram powder

2 tsp paprika

Directions:

1. Preheat grill to a medium heat.
2. In a bowl, mix the cumin, marjoram, paprika, garlic, olive oil, lime juice, coriander, and hot sauce.
3. Season the tuna steaks with sea salt and black pepper.
4. Coat the seasoned tuna steaks with the coriander-lime sauce.
5. Place the tuna on the grill.
6. Cook 4 minutes per side till the pinkish hue is gone.
7. Let it rest a few minutes before serving.

Authentic Chinese Shrimp

Ingredients:

2 tbsp ginger, shredded

4 tbsp coconut oil

2 tbsp cornstarch

4 tbsp cold water

2 tsp rice wine vinegar

2 tsp lime juice

2 tsp raw honey

30 medium shrimps, peeled and deveined

2 onion, chopped

2 red bell pepper, diced

6 red chilies, dried

2 garlic clove, minced

Fresh parsley

Directions:

1. In a bowl, mix cornstarch, apple cider vinegar, lime juice, honey, and water.
2. Melt the coconut oil in a pan over a medium heat. Add the ginger and garlic, frying till it is fragrant.
3. Add the onion, bell pepper, and red chilies to the pan. Cook until onions are transparent.
4. Place the shrimps in the skillet. Cook until it turns pink.
5. Pour in the lime blend. Stir well.
6. Cook until the sauce simmers to preferred consistency.
7. Serve topped with fresh parsley.

Aztec Fish Stew

Ingredients:

2 garlic cloves, chopped

4 tbsp lime juice

4 tbsp cumin powder

2 tbsp paprika

2 tsp cayenne pepper

2 cups coconut milk

2 cups vegetable stock

2 lb cod, cut into bite-sized bits

2 red bell pepper, diced

2 yellow bell pepper, diced

2 onion, minced

4 tbsp olive oil

Coconut oil

Sea salt and pepper

Directions:

1. In a bowl, mix the lime juice, olive oil, salt, and pepper.
2. Add the fish. Flip until well coated.
3. Heat some coconut oil in a large skillet over a medium-high heat.
4. Add the garlic, onion, and bell peppers. Cook until tender.
5. Pour in the vegetable stock and coconut milk. Let simmer for a minute.
6. Add in the cumin, paprika, and cayenne.
7. Bring the soup to a boil, then lower the heat to a simmer. Add the fish to the broth.
8. Cover the stew. Cook until the fish flakes.
9. Serve the stew hot with lime wedges.

Jamaican Ribs

Ingredients:

2 lb spare ribs

Seasoning:

2 tsp black pepper

1 tsp cinnamon

1 tsp nutmeg

2 tsp paprika

2 tsp cayenne pepper

2 tbsp onion, minced

2 tsp dried thyme

2 tsp allspice

Sea salt

Sauce:

2 tsp lime zest

4 tbsp lime juice

2 tbsp cornstarch

2 tsp ginger, minced

2 garlic cloves, minced

2 cup Paleo ketchup

1/2 cup apple juice

2 tbsp raw honey

Directions:

1. Preheat the oven to 4 30 ºF.
2. Mix all seasoning ingredients. Rub the ribs uniformly with most of the seasoning.

Leave about a quarter of the seasoning for later.
3. Cover the ribs and bake in the oven for 4 hours.
4. Mix all the ingredients for the sauce in a small pan with the remaining seasoning over a medium heat.
5. Simmer until thickened.
6. Remove from heat. Let the sauce cool down.
7. Preheat grill to medium-high heat.
8. Baste all the ribs liberally with the sauce. Place on the grill.
9. Grill the ribs 30 minutes, basting with sauce every 10 minutes.

Crackling Pork Chili

Ingredients:

4 cups canned tomatoes

1/2 cup chili powder

2 tbsp paprika

2 tbsp cumin

1/2 tsp cayenne pepper

4 tbsp red wine vinegar

4 lbs pork shoulder

2 onions, sliced

2 red chilis, chopped

2 bell peppers, sliced

4 garlic cloves, minced

1/2 cup olive oil

Fresh oregano leaves, minced

Sea salt and pepper

Directions:

1. Preheat the oven to 4 6 0ºF.
2. Warm the olive oil in an oven-safe stew pot over a medium heat, add the garlic, onions, and red chilies. Cook for 6 minutes or until the onions are soft.
3. Lower the heat. Add the bell peppers, tomatoes, chili powder, paprika, cumin, cayenne pepper, oregano leaves, salt, and pepper.
4. Place the pork shoulder in the pot, and stir well. Trickle in the red wine vinegar. Pour in enough water to submerge the meat.
5. Bring to a simmer, cover, and place in the oven for 4 1 hours.
6. Serve hot.

Bigos

Ingredients:

2 lb sausage, preferably kielbasa, sliced

2 onions, diced

2 cloves garlic, minced

2 bay leaf

Grass-fed cow's butter

Sea salt and pepper

2 cup cabbage, washed and sliced

4 cups sauerkraut

2 can tomato paste

2 lb bacon, cut into bits

1 lb pork, diced

Directions:

1. In a shallow bottomed pan, boil the sliced cabbage till tender.
2. In a separate pot, boil the sauerkraut in about one and a half cups of water. Strain and keep the sour water aside for future use.
3. Stir-fry the pork in a pan with some butter. Then set aside.
4. Fry the bacon and sausage with the onion and garlic.
5. In a large pot, mix the cooked cabbage, sauerkraut, sour water, tomato paste, spices, meats, onion, and garlic.
6. Let simmer for about 2 hour. Serve warm.

Butter Chicken

Ingredients:

2 tsp ground coriander

2 tbsp fresh ginger, grated

1 chili powder

2 cinnamon stick

6 cardamom pods

2 cup tomato purée

¾ cup coconut milk

4 tbsp grass-fed cow's butter

2 lbs chicken, cut into uniform pieces

2 1 tsp garam masala

2 tsp paprika

2 tbsp fresh lemon juice

Fresh coriander leaves, chopped

Directions:

1. Heat a heavy-bottomed pan, add half of the butter, and sauté the chicken. When the chicken is cooked through, remove from the pan and set aside.
2. Add the rest of the butter and, on the lowest temperature, sauté the garam masala, paprika, coriander, ginger, chili powder, cinnamon, and cardamom pods for a minute or two until fragrant.
3. Put the chicken back in the pan with the spices and stir well to coat the meat with the spices.
4. Pour in the tomatoes. Cook for about 30 minutes. Stir occasionally.
5. Add the coconut milk and lemon juice. Let it boil for another 10 minutes.
6. Sprinkle chopped coriander leaves. Serve hot with cauliflower rice.

Taro Chips

Ingredients:

2 tbsp olive oil

Sea salt and pepper

2 lbs taro roots, rinsed and peeled

Directions:

1. Preheat the oven to 4 6 0ºF.
2. Using a sharp knife, cut the taro root into slim rounds no thicker than a quarter of an inch.
3. Add the sliced taro roots and olive oil in a bowl. Flip the bowl to coat lightly.
4. Arrange the taro root slices in a single layer on a greased baking sheet.
5. Season with salt and pepper.

6. Place in the oven and bake for 4 0 minutes, turning halfway through, until they are golden brown and crisp.

Salt Crackers

Ingredients:

2 fresh Eggs , large

Sea salt and pepper

4 cups almond flour

Directions:

1. Add in the almond flour, egg, salt, and pepper in a bowl.
2. Knead well until a solid dough is created.

3. Set dough between 2 pieces of parchment paper.
4. Using slight pressure, roll out the dough to 2 /8 inch thickness, then remove the parchment paper on top.
5. Carefully, transfer the parchment paper with rolled out dough onto a baking tray.
6. Using a butter knife, cut into 2-inch squares.
7. Adjust seasoning, if desired.
8. Bake at 4 6 0ºF for 30 minutes.
9. Seal in an airtight jar after cooling down.

Bengali Almonds

Ingredients:

- 2 tbsp coconut oil
- 4 cups almonds
- ¾ tsp turmeric

- 1/2 tsp cumin
  1/2 tsp coriander
  Sea salt and pepper

Directions:

1. Add the coconut oil in a shallow-bottomed pan over a medium heat. Do not let the oil smoke or fume.
2. Add almonds to the oil.
3. After toasting the almonds for a minute, mix in salt, turmeric, pepper, cumin, and coriander.
4. Continue toasting for about five more minutes.
5. Take off the heat. Allow the almonds to cool.
6. Place in an airtight jar and store in a cool place.

The James' Secret Dill Pickles

Ingredients:

2 cayenne pepper pod

4 tbsp dill, fresh, chopped

4 cups cold water

Sea salt

30 gherkin cucumbers, rinsed

4 cloves garlic, halved

4 bay leaves

Directions:

1. Arrange the gherkins in a spacious wide-mouthed jar.
2. Toss in the garlic, bay leaves, cayenne pod, and dill in the jar with the cucumbers.
3. Seal the jar tightly. Shake well. Set aside.
4. Mix salt and cold water together.
5. Fill up the jar to the brim with the salt water.
6. Seal the jar and store in a cool place for a week.
7. Store in the refrigerator after opening. Use only dry utensils when fishing out the gherkins.

Vermont Sweet Pecans

Ingredients:

2 tbsp ghee

4 tbsp maple syrup

Sea salt

2 cups pecans

Directions:

1. Add all ingredients together in a large bowl. Stir well to fuse all flavors together.
2. Place on a greased baking tray.
3. Bake at 4 6 0ºF for 30 minutes.
4. Cool and store in an airtight jar.

www.ingramcontent.com/pod-product-compliance
Lightning Source LLC
LaVergne TN
LVHW011938070526
838202LV00054B/4703